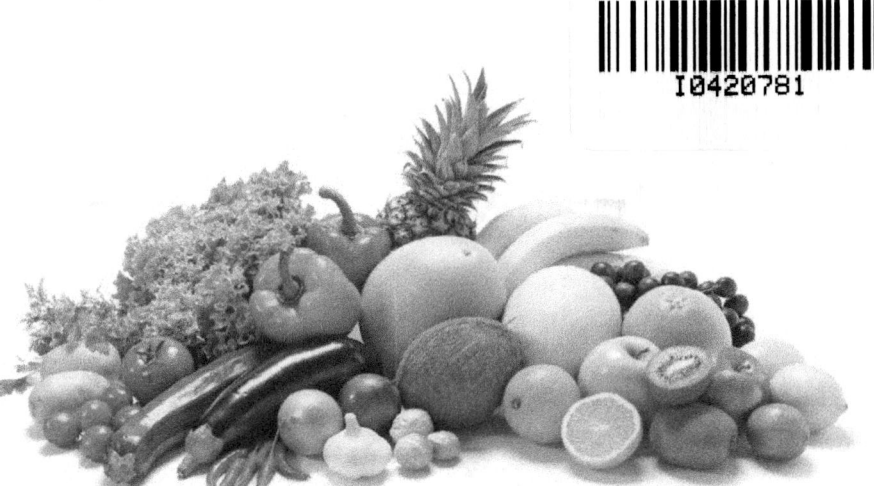

Rejuvenate Your Health

With 8 Simple Steps

" Good Health is not being a certain size.
It's a lifestyle of making healthy decisions
that benefit the Mind, Body, & Spirit. "
~ Coach Denise

Denise Simpson, CHHP, AADP

Foreword by Hazel Dixon-Cooper

Thank you for purchasing this Book!

Please visit my website to Join the My Life Healthy mailing list and receive health tips, recipes, and so much more.

www.MyLifeHealthy.com

Notice: This book is not intended to replace recommendations or advice from physicians or other healthcare providers. Rather, it is intended to help you make informed decisions about your health and to cooperate with your healthcare provider in a joint quest for optimal wellness. If you suspect you have a medical problem, we urge you to seek medical attention from a competent healthcare provider.

My Life Healthy With Denise, LLC
Post Office Box 5361
Tallahassee, Fl 32314
http://www.MyLifeHealthy.com

This book is dedicated to all who desire a higher level of health and wellness. The body is a complex system. Your body will respond to how you treat it whether good or bad. Be sure to take good care of your body. You only get one!

Table of Contents

Acknowledgments

I owe a great many thanks to many people who helped and supported me during the writing of this book.

My deepest love and appreciation goes to my husband of over 30 years, Dennis. Thank you for supporting me and allowing me to soar. You make my life complete.

To my children and grandchildren, I hope you are inspired to release your potential and pursue your purpose. Greatness is all I see in you!

I would especially like to thank my good friend Delores. Words cannot express what you mean to my life and my family. Your wisdom is astute! Good "brain" food.

To the late Dr. Myles Munroe, I am forever grateful for your teachings, your passion for the student learner, and your profound kingdom wisdom. Thank you for challenging me to become greater – Pursuing Purpose.

Foreword

Sometimes the simplest steps are the hardest to take. I wish I'd had Denise Simpson's book one hundred pounds ago. Back then, I had an excuse for everything I ate and a long list of reasons why I could not get off my butt and exercise.

Like you, I had great intentions, but in spite of those intentions, I repeatedly stuffed myself to the brink of illness, especially during the holidays. Then repenting like a Saturday-night sinner at a Sunday-morning revival meeting, I rushed to the nearest gym or joined the latest lose-it-quick weight-loss program. Sound familiar?

But after a couple of weeks, and just as you begin to feel human again, Super Bowl Sunday roars up the driveway, tailgate flapping, loaded with hot wings, stuffed jalapenos and supermarket meat-and-cheese platters. Any thought of healthy eating ends with the first mouthful of chili-cheese dip.

Oh well, it's only one day.

Before you wipe the last smear of wing sauce off your face, oops, here comes Valentine's Day. Break out the chocolate and champagne. By the time you pick the caramel out of your teeth, St. Patrick swings by with a heaping helping of corned beef, cabbage, and green beer. Right on his heels, Easter drags in a basketful of chocolate bunnies. Before the dye dries on the eggs, Mother's Day rings the doorbell. You take Mom out for a calorie-loaded dinner that is sure to raise both her cholesterol and her blood pressure. Yours too. But no worries. It's only one day.

Memorial Day kick-starts summer with the first official barbecue of the season. Father's Day is next on the menu. All Dad wants to do is flop in front of the sports channel and eat, and you are happy to accommodate him. Spread out the food on the coffee table, wrap a beach towel around his neck, and let him chomp himself into a heart attack. Hope the life insurance is paid up.

Summer appears with a bang on the Fourth of July, another grilling-and-chilling holiday. Mid-July through August is vacation time, and who counts calories at the beach? Instead, you tell yourself that is the only time you can truly relax, so you gladly live on sugar, carbs, and fat-laden non-food. Besides, you deserve to indulge. Right?

As soon you are home, Labor Day weekend and the last binge of the season arrive. When the kids head back to school, you head, credit card in hand, to the nearest diet center or gym. That lasts about four weeks, until Halloween creeps in again. You have come full circle and are about to take another trip into the Bermuda Triangle of holiday food benders.

Add to this list Hanukkah, Eid-ul-fitr, Kwanzaa, and a multitude of other religious or spiritual festivities, weddings, showers, anniversaries, birthdays, funerals, Sunday dinners, and other personal celebrations. The result? Out of a 52-two week year, most people resolve to lose weight the week after New Year's and the week after Labor Day. Think about it. Two weeks out of an entire year. Isn't your health worth more than that?

According to the U.S. Surgeon General, 300,000 people a year die prematurely from obesity-related diseases. Saying no to Aunt Fanny's banana pudding cake or Uncle Ralph's roasted beast with mango chutney is tough. We've all heard, "I made this just for you," accompanied by a hurt expression. Out of guilt, and an ever-present craving, you eat the casserole or cake or candy. If you decline, they counter with, "It's only one day."

What can you do?

Well, you can continue to eat anything that anyone shoves your way and risk turning into an insulin-shooting diabetic stumbling around on your last three toes. You could eat yourself into a case of dementia, or be diagnosed with late-stage cancer because the fat hid the tumor.

Or you can begin to get healthy. One skipped order of French fries, one refused dessert, one trade from fried chicken to grilled halibut will start to turn your life and your health in the right direction. That's how I lost one hundred pounds. One bite, one choice, one day at a time.

And you have the help that I didn't. You can learn Coach Denise's eight simple steps to rejuvenating your health, starting right now.

Hazel Dixon-Cooper is an internationally best-selling author and former columnist for Cosmopolitan magazine. She is currently working on a memoir, CONFESSIONS OF A FAT COSMO GIRL, and can be reached at hazeldixon.cooper@gmail.com.

Introduction

Obesity has rapidly turned into a global concern. Studies show that in 2014, the top 5 most obese countries were the United States, China, India, Russia, and Brazil with Mexico at number six. As the obesity epidemic continues to increase, so does heart disease, diabetes, and cancer which are claiming more lives each year. Statistics show that incidences of these diseases are much higher now than half a century ago. The obsessive struggle between fast food and whole food is real. Why is it that there is a sharp deterioration in human health?

Well, it's simple! Food is the common denominator for mostly everything we do on a daily bases. Whether leaving the workplace to grab lunch, or meeting at a restaurant to discuss a business deal, or attending a social gathering - it all involves food. People in general are usually not thinking about or paying attention to calories consumed, recommended servings, or the quality of their food, only whether it tastes good, is reasonably priced and if the environment is good.

The quality of our food has taken a downward turn since the early 1900's. Our food today is usually grown in nutrient depleted soils, resulting from overuse, making the quality of our fruits and vegetables low grade. Our food is laden with pesticides, preservatives and other chemicals. There are questionable regulations that govern the safety of our food. With the increased use of additives, fillers, and other ways to bulk up our food – most of what we eat is not real food.

Another factor, the modern lifestyle creates workaholics who deprive themselves of needed rest and good nutrition. People are so busy working to attain esteemed living that they are sacrificing their health. This along with poor eating habits and lack of exercise creates stress within the body and later stress-related illnesses such as heart disease, asthma, obesity and gastrointestinal problems to name a few. Most people have not made the connection that good health is tied to their happiness and overall wellbeing.

A sad fact is that a majority of people know exactly what they need to do when it comes to improving their health, but they simply choose to do otherwise. In most cases, people only need a will to improve and someone to help them be accountable, at least starting off. Accountability will help you stay the course long enough to allow you to change your habits. Let's be honest here. Why do you think so many people falter with their New Year's resolutions? It's because people give way on their goals by letting themselves off the hook. Accountability brings results!

Rejuvenate Your Health was pinned to show you simple ways to slim down, regain energy, and bring back a more youthful vibrant energetic you! By changing your eating habits, increasing your movement throughout the day, and engaging in more self-care, you can expect to have increased energy levels, alertness, and feel more balanced as you move toward achieving your ideal wellness goals.

And by all means, seek the assistance of a health and wellness coach to support you on your journey. Age is only a number, seriously! It should not determine how you look and feel. Walk with me through this book to learn how you can give your health a new lifeline by incorporating these eight simple steps.

Chapter 1: Drink More Water

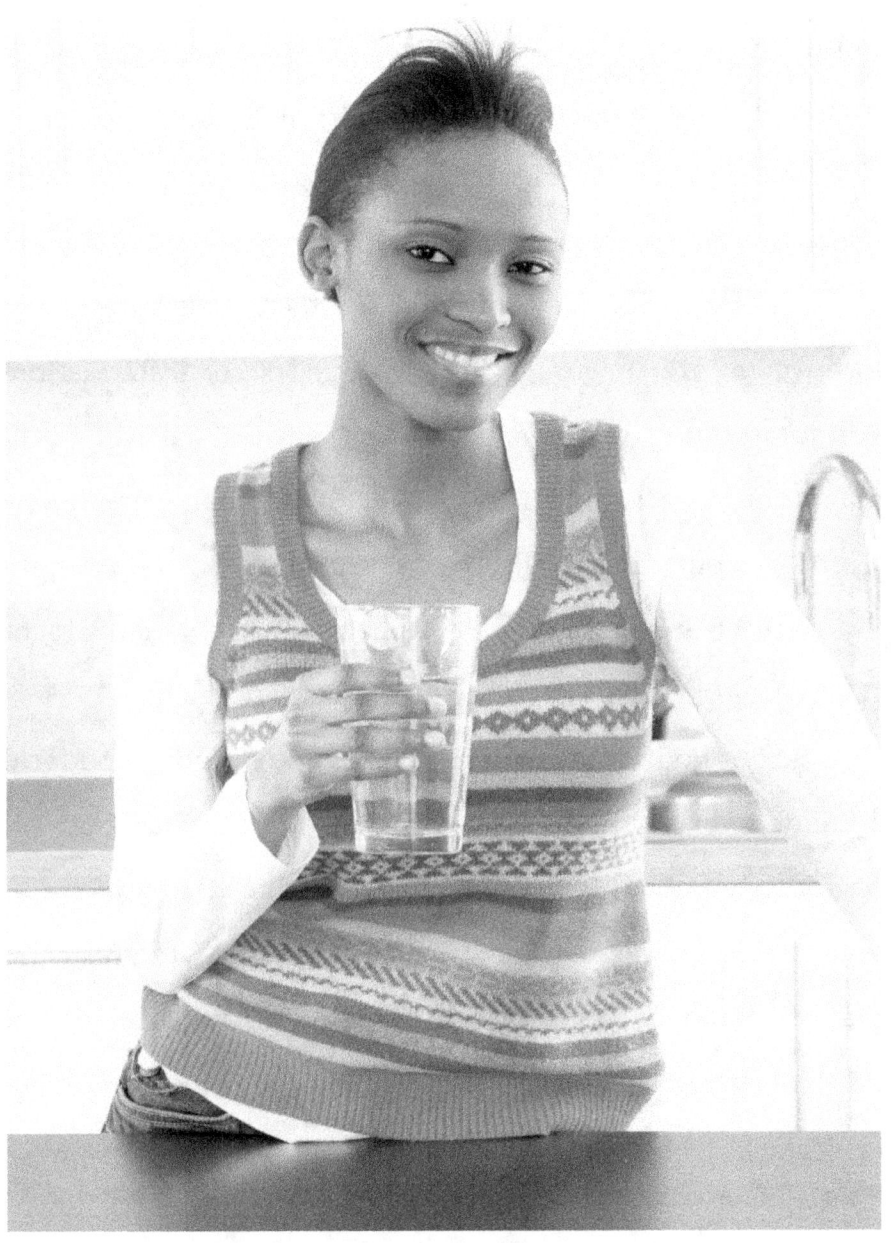

Drink More Water

Water and good health walk hand in hand. Although most Americans have realized the need to constantly stay hydrated, not enough of us do so. The old eight-glasses-a-day rule had no scientific backing but was a guide to encourage people to drink more water. We need more now.

Many people who often watch their diets in a bid to lose weight are encouraged to consume lots of water. Before you jump out of your skin thinking that drinking water will make you lose weight faster, understand that water alone won't be your magic pill. The relevance of water to weight loss comes from the fact that it can be used to replace the high-calorie beverages partly responsible for weight gain.

Your body is in constant need of body fluids to perform a number of functions. As you may know, your body is composed of about 70 percent water. Reduce the intake, and you can suffer serious fluid imbalance. So drink the water so that you can help digestion, saliva, excretion, transportation of nutrients, absorption, and other functions in the body.

Key Role in Detoxification

Water also plays a major role in the body's detoxification process. One part of the body that relies on adequate water intake is the kidneys. Water is crucial for the proper functioning of the kidneys, which are essentially the body's detoxification machine. The kidneys are organs that might not get as much attention as the heart or lungs, but they are responsible for many functions that help keep the body as healthy as possible.

A crucial function of the kidneys is to remove waste products and excess fluid from the body via urine. The kidneys also regulate the levels of salt, potassium and acid in the body and produce hormones that influence the performance of other organs. Most of the toxins that pass through the kidney are soluble in water, and when you have enough fluids in the body, you increase the amount of toxins that get expelled via urine.

That is why whenever you take in lots of water, you go for short calls quite often, and you pass colorless and odorless urine. But when you don't drink enough water, urination becomes less frequent and you pass concentrated urine that is darker in color and has a strong odor associated with it. The difference between the two situations is the magic brought about by drinking enough water.

How Much Water Should You Drink?

The earlier campaign of drinking eight glasses a day has been refuted, but this does not mean you should reduce your intake. On the contrary, drink as much water as you can, and never allow yourself to get thirsty. A good rule of thumb is to drink half your body weight in water every day. To explain, if you weigh 150 pounds, divide that number in half and drink that amount in ounces. In this case, it would be 75 ounces per day which is equivalent to about 9 cups of water. This should be enough to keep you well hydrated.

Although that may seem like a lot and likely to cause several unscheduled visits to restroom, after several days the body will adjust and you will love how you feel. Thirst comes when the water levels in your body have reduced significantly, and the hypothalamus section of your brain sends a distress signal to the pituitary glands. By this time, the damage is already done, so never let yourself get thirsty. Take it literally—water is life. The more you drink, the more alive you become.

What is the Best Water to Drink?

Who would have ever imagined that something as simple as drinking water could become so complicated. Today, we have bottled water in a number of varieties. From the type of water – distilled, spring water, purified water, vitamin water, osmosis water – to the brand of water.

My approach to selecting water as well as food has been to choose what is most natural, less invasive, and simple. For me, I shy away from purchasing bottled water as much as possible for a number of reasons. In the general sense, bottled water has been known to carry more toxins than your regular tap water from the faucet. Claims from where the water comes from to fill the bottles is questionable.

I remember reading an article where bottled water was known to carry more than 24,500 chemicals with one being BPA (bisphenol-A). BPA is a common chemical used to make plastic bottles and linings of cans. Studies show that under certain temperature this chemical may seep into the water. Recently, the Food and Drug Administration (FDA) banned the use of BPA in making plastic.

What is most practical is to invest in a reusable BPA-free water bottle. Choosing bottles made of nontoxic glass or stainless steel is highly recommended to ensure your health and safety. As for the actual water, using a typical homemade water filter or portable water filter to purify your tap water will save you time and money in the long run.

Drinking water is like washing out your insides. The water will cleanse the system, fill you up, decrease your caloric load and improve the function of all your tissues.

~ Kevin R. Stone

Chapter 2: Eat Whole Foods

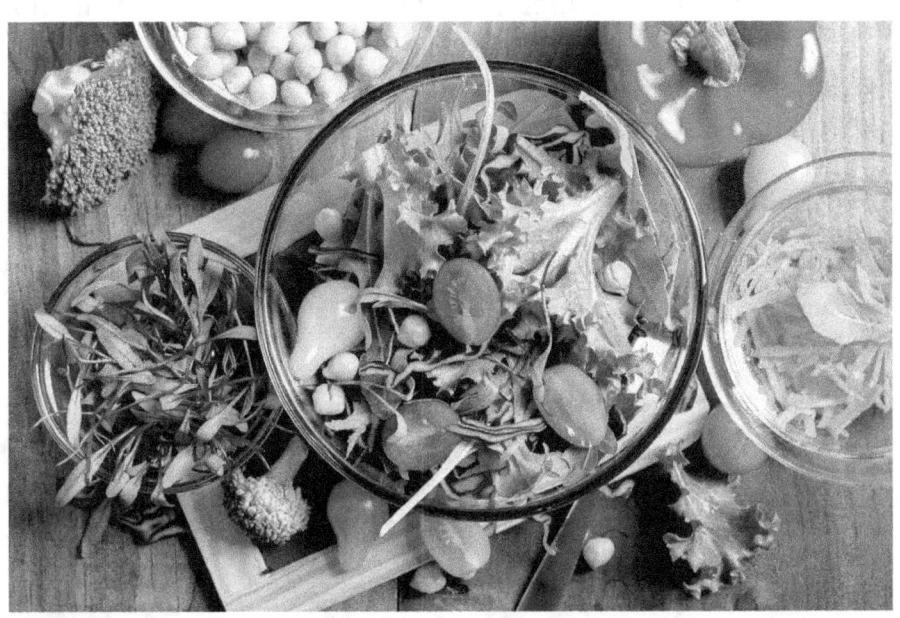

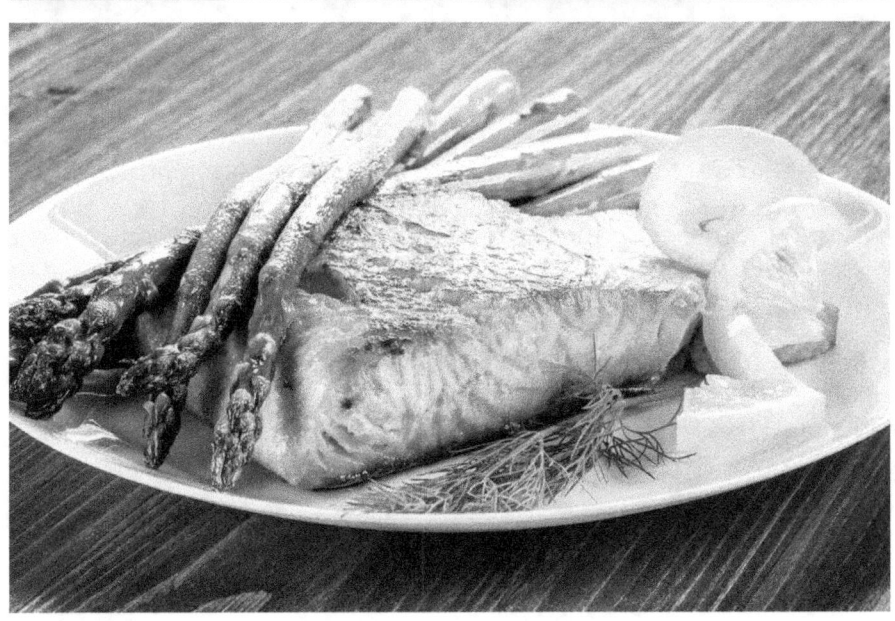

Eat Whole Foods

Our modern lifestyle has made it difficult if not impossible for a majority of people to find time to prepare healthy meals with proper nutritional benefits. Queues in fast-food joints are always full as people find the most convenient foods instead of preparing their own meals at home. It is disturbing that most people who go for the fast food already understand the inherent health consequences of consuming such junk. Yet they ignore the warnings.

Fast foods and processed foods in the general sense are the culprits in causing the body to become toxic, which later result in ailments that are commonly referred to as lifestyle diseases. If only people would gravitate towards eating more whole foods – foods in its natural state (fresh vegetables, fruit, whole grains, organic proteins), Americans wouldn't be laboring with back-breaking medical bills to maintain diabetes, heart conditions, and kidney problems among others.

Avoid Processed Foods

Although processed foods might be appealing to the eye and tempting to the taste buds, they carry with them serious health consequences. During the processing of these foods, vital components that are essential to the body are extracted and replaced with additives and preservatives that have zero nutritional benefits. These foods come loaded with artery-clogging substances such as cholesterol, which is the main cause of heart disease and ultimately heart failure.

It is also important to observe that most people who love processed foods are the ones who suffer the most from obesity and weight-related problems. Processed foods are foods high in calories that spike your insulin levels and trigger the body into "fat storage" mode. What this means is that your fat cells expand and so does your clothing size over time. Most soft drinks deposit bad sugars into the system, and these sugars later culminate into various types of diabetes. In short, processed food does nothing but cause more misery to the body, and it has no relevance to human health as far as proper nutrition is concerned.

Why Switch?

Whole foods, on the other hand, have all the nutritional requirements that are not only necessary for good health, but also for enhancing the immune system thus preventing many diseases. You might be asking what are whole foods. Whole foods consist of foods that are grown naturally with minimal processing, alterations, and are how nature designed them.

These foods consist mainly of fruits, vegetables, and whole grains like quinoa, buckwheat, amaranth, bulgur, and brown rice to name a few. They are referred to as whole foods because they haven't undergone any form of processing, and they still have their maximum nutritional components. Before you walk back into your favorite fast-food restaurant or you stuff your shopping cart at the supermarket with a variety of processed foods from the freezer, consider the following benefits that you will be missing from whole foods.

- Phytonutrients. These powerful nutrients are responsible for fighting free radicals present in the atmosphere that might cause harm when they get into the body. In most cases, the free radicals react with the elements found in the skin to form wrinkles and to reduce the skin's ability to offer protection against the harmful ultraviolet rays of the sun. Dietary fiber. Fruits, whole grains, and vegetables are rich in dietary fiber, which is essential in weight loss and reduction of cholesterol in the body. The fiber replaces bad fats that would normally be deposited under the skin and in turn encourages muscle development. They also carry enzymes that are good for digestion.

- Disease-fighting vitamins and nutrients. These vitamins and nutrients enhance the body's immune system, thus offering protection from most of the common ailments. These foods can also reduce the occurrence of some of the most life-threatening lifestyle diseases, including diabetes, stroke, and heart diseases, and they are also super effective in weight management.

Now that you have the facts about both processed and whole foods, make a conscious decision to choose the path to heal your body. When your eating habits improve, so will your health. There is a saying: "Let your food be your medicine." There are healing properties in whole foods just the way nature intended. When the body is supplied with proper nutrients it begins to thrive! Can you imagine having no joint pain, no brain fog or irritability, renewed energy and much more? Expect all of these benefits after you clean up your diet.

It's better to get the nutrients for healthy skin from food, not supplements. Salmon, walnuts, blueberries, spinach... lots of my favorite foods happen to be amazing for skin too.

~ Gail Simmons

Chapter 3: Stop Skipping Breakfast

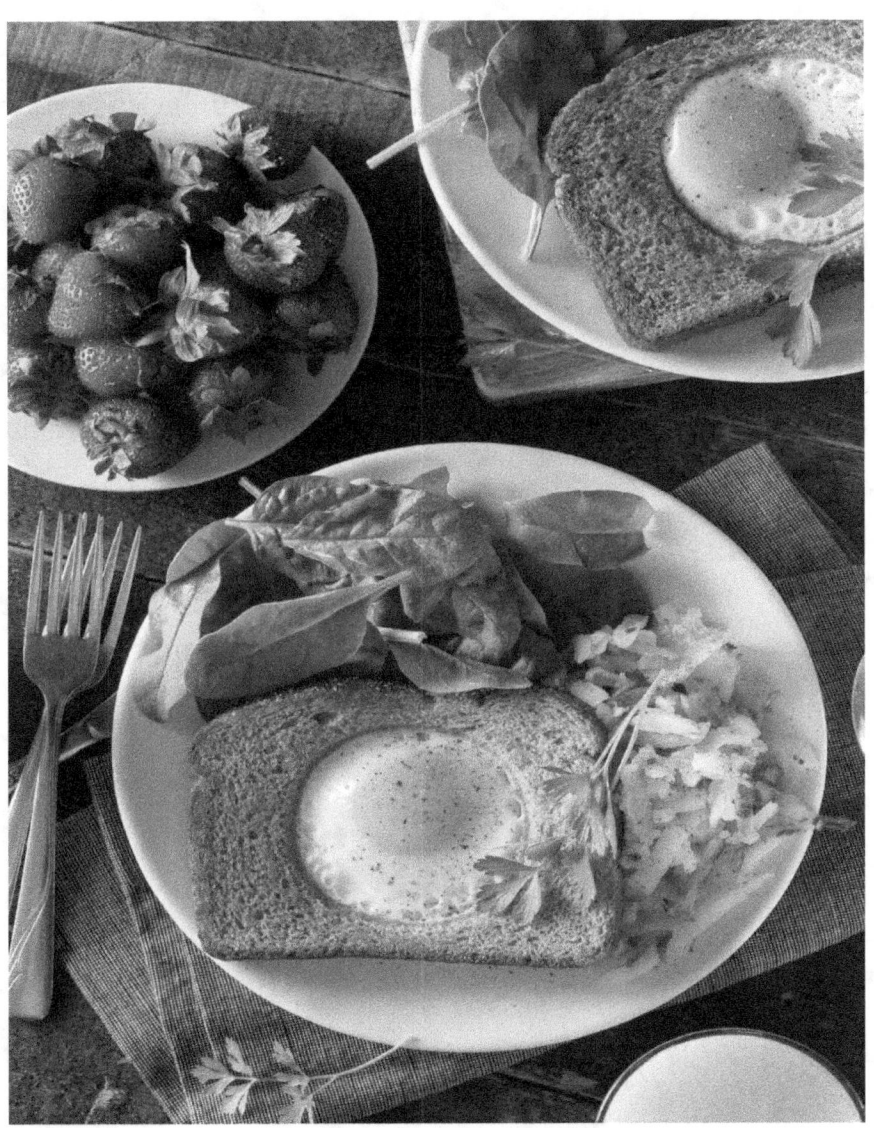

You have probably heard that breakfast is the most important meal of the day. This is not just a cliché. There are valid reasons why you should not skip breakfast. The simple explanation is that when you skip breakfast you develop a tendency to snack more, which does nothing but increase your daily calorie intake. Also, studies show that many overweight people who skip breakfast binge late at night. As a result, they create a cycle for themselves of skipping breakfast, followed by snacking, overeating, and binging. Several researchers have associated the following lapses in daily performances as a result of doing so.

- Reduced physical activity
- Poor concentration
- Weakened ability to solve problems expediently
- Poor eye-hand coordination

Importance of a healthy breakfast every morning

However busy your morning schedule might be, you should start the day with good nutrition. Eating a nutritional breakfast will not only give you a head start for the day's energy requirements, but it will also provide you with marvelous health benefits that have been associated with weight loss and peak performance. Eating protein for breakfast such as eggs, quinoa, tofu, yogurt, nuts and seeds, or meat will allow you to feel full for most of the morning and you won't feel like snacking. You will also have a reduced desire to binge at lunchtime as opposed to when you miss breakfast and are tempted to "compensate" at lunch.

Other than helping you lose weight, a healthy breakfast will give you the right energy boost in the morning. During the night, while you're sleeping, you spend energy sustaining the basal metabolic rate. In this process, energy is used, which in turn depletes the glucose levels in the body. You wake up with a deficiency in your glucose levels that will affect your energy levels, alertness, as well as your moods throughout the day. The result is a reduction in your efficiency in accomplishing various tasks. But a nutritious breakfast will replenish the energy reserves and put you in the right mood to face each day with optimism.

To keep your metabolism running at full capacity, meaning you are always in a state of thermogenesis, you need to eat regular, frequent meals. Studies show that eating breakfast can increase your resting metabolism by up to 10 percent. In order to reap maximum benefits from this important morning meal, you need to make careful choices. Ideally, a healthy breakfast is comprised of whole grains, lean proteins, fresh fruit juices, and vegetables. Unless you incorporate most of these in your morning meal, you will have missed the whole point of eating breakfast.

Simple ideas for a healthy breakfast meal

Here are a few breakfast ideas that require little preparation time and offer good health benefits.

- Smoothies made from fresh fruits and vegetables
- Plain Greek yogurt, fruit, and flaxseed
- A bowl of quinoa topped with fruit and nuts or made as a porridge
- Scrambled eggs, tomato slices together with whole wheat English muffin
- Oatmeal prepared with skim milk, nuts, and raisins served with fresh orange juice.

Now take it upon yourself to search for more healthful and quick breakfast ideas so that you can have a variety of options. This will ensure that whatever you consume for breakfast will provide the energy you need to sustain you throughout the day.

Breakfast is the most important meal of the day. When you feed yourself what your body needs when it needs it, that's love. So give your bod some TLC and sit down and enjoy a good, substantial breakfast.

~Kathy Freston

Chapter Four: Eat Healthy Fats

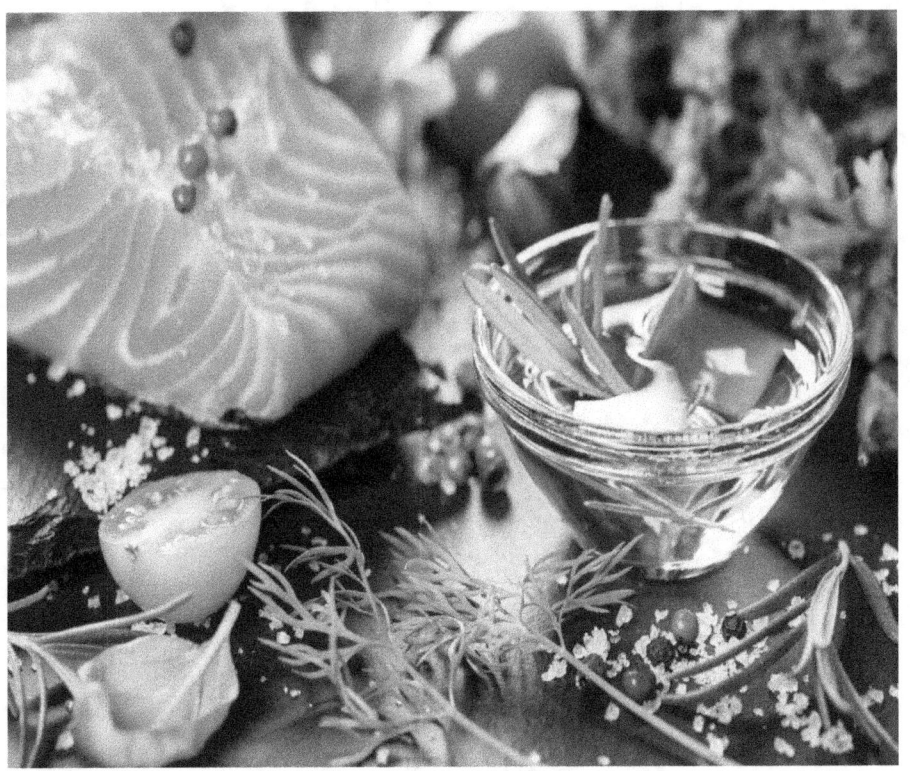

For many years, a majority of people have associated fats to heart conditions and weight gain. Although this notion might hold water in some instances, it should not be taken that all fats are bad and should be avoided. There is great need for people to understand the difference between bad fats and good fats so that they can make a distinction between the two whenever they are making their health purchases.

Understanding dietary fats

You may have probably taken note of some products at the grocery store—ice cream and candy, for instance—that claim to be low- or non-fat food. The problem with such products is that when they are consumed, people still go ahead and gain weight and also risk heart disease. In short, these foods may not be as healthy as they pretend.

There is a difference between good fats and bad fats. Bad fats are basically comprised of trans fats and saturated fats, and they are the ones responsible for weight gain, clogging the arteries, heart diseases, and cancer. Good fats, on the other hand, consist of monounsaturated fats and polyunsaturated fats. These are responsible for myriad health benefits.

- They deliver fat-soluble vitamins to the body.

- They are instant sources of energy.

- They improve mental health.

- They help fight fatigue.

- They control weight gain.

Bad fats and their sources

If you want to stop risking your heart and exposing yourself to various types of cancer, then you must do away with Trans fats and saturated fats. Trans fats come from the hydrogenation of vegetable oils so as to make it more stable and enable it to last long. This is good for the manufacturers but detrimental to your health. The common sources of these fats include baked foods, friend foods, snacks, and solid fats.

Saturated fats are found from animal products and whole-milk dairy products. Fish and poultry products may at times contain this type of fat but in lesser quantities as compared to products like red meat. Their common sources include butter, cheese, cream, whole milk, cream, and red meat.

Get more good fats into your system

Now that you understand the sources of bad fats and how they affect the body, it is important to replace them with the monounsaturated and polyunsaturated fats. You can achieve this by doing the following.

- Use olive oil or coconut oil for cooking instead of butter or stick margarine and use vegetable oils for baking.

- Eat more avocadoes. Healthy for the brain and the heart, they are extremely satisfying.

- Eat nuts and seeds such as walnuts, almonds, pecans; pumpkin, flax and hemp seeds.

- Avoid commercials salads. Instead make your own healthy ones by using cold pressed olive oils, sesame oils, or flaxseed oils.

Super fats for the brain and heart: Omega 3 fatty acids

Omega 3 fatty acids are types of polyunsaturated fats, and even though these and the monounsaturated fats are good for the health, omega 3 fatty acids are extremely beneficial for brain and heart health. The major sources of omega 3 are fish, and the best ones are salmon, sardines, mackerel, tuna, and lake trout. The following are some of the particular benefits of omega 3 fatty acids.

- They significantly reduce the risk of heart disease, cancer, and stroke.
- They guard against memory loss, thus offering protection against dementia.
- They support healthy pregnancy.
- They ease joint pain and inflammation.
- They reduce or prevent depression.

There you have it! Adjust your diet accordingly. Replace your sources of bad fats with polyunsaturated and monounsaturated fats so that you stay safe from some of the deadliest lifestyle diseases.

Certainly adding fats in the form of oils is fattening and unhealthy, but naturally fat-rich foods like nuts and seeds have profound cardiovascular benefits.

~ Joel Fuhrman

Chapter Five: Exercise Regularly

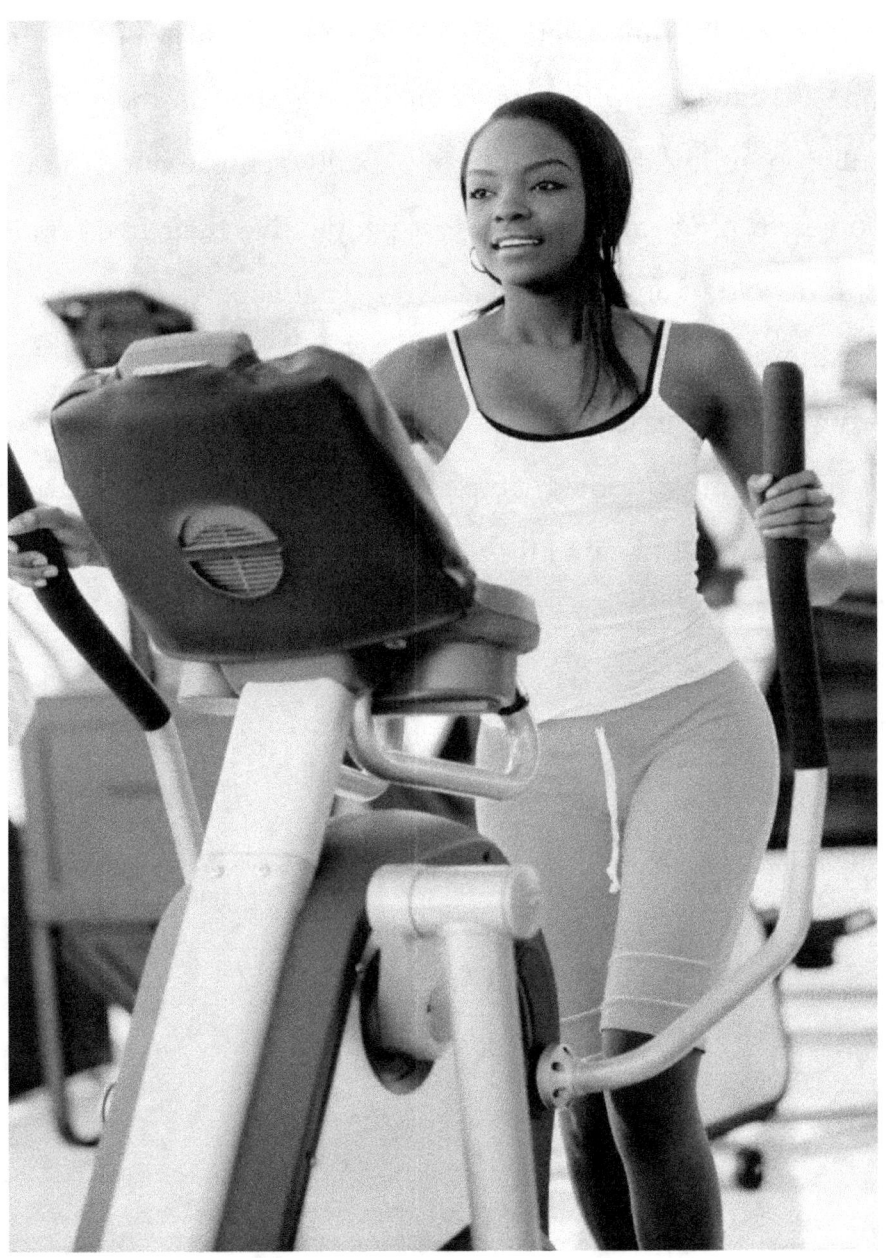

Staying active by exercising regularly and observing a healthy diet is what most physicians and nutritionists recommend as the prerequisites for good health. But at the present time, people seem to have forgotten the benefits of fully observing the two, and they totally get it wrong when it comes to physical activity. Most people live their lives static and devoid of any physical activity. That is part of the reason for the significant increase in the number of people suffering from heart disease, diabetes, arthritis, stress, and depression. If people only adopted simple health regimens on a regular basis, they would gain huge health benefits.

The cost of inactivity

A classic example of being inactive is to sit for long hours either working on the computer or watching television with snacks in your hands. Researches done by several institutions have associated such levels of inactivity to increased weight gain and risks of getting diabetes. Studies have also suggested that those who stay put for a long time have increased chances of getting cardiovascular diseases. As a result, such people have a higher likelihood to spend more on health care than those who stay active in their lives.

There are certain little changes that anyone can introduce to their lives to reverse being inactive and prevent a myriad of health complications. For instance, deciding to go three floors up by the stairs rather than using the escalators or elevator can perform real magic in your life. Also deciding to take a walk around the neighborhood instead of sitting for hours playing games on the computer or watching television will also go a long way in introducing some form of physical activity into your life.

Health Benefits of exercise

There is no arguing that exercise is important in anyone's health only that people tend to ignore it with the pretext of being busy. Fortunately, there are a number of different types of effective exercises that can be performed on a regular basis without having to go visit the gym or pay any subscription fees to a health club. Laziness and ignorance are thus the main things that deter people from utilizing exercises to improve their health. The following are some of the health benefits of regular exercises-:

- Weight management – physical activities done during exercising burn a lot of calories and this can be beneficial to someone who has excessive weight and would love to shed off some.

- Improves health conditions and prevents diseases – regular exercises will reduce the levels of bad cholesterol in your body and as a result, you will have improved cardiovascular health. Besides, regular physical activity will enhance your moods, lower stress and reduce the instances of being attacked by depression.

- Energy boost – physical activity will lead to the development of better, stronger and healthier muscles. You will also give a lot of resilience to your muscles tissues as well as making your heart and lungs work much better. This will give you the energy required to perform most of the normal chores.

- Lowers high blood pressure – during physical activity, there is an increase in the heart rate. This in turn enhances the body's ability to utilize oxygen thus ensuring optimum blood pressure.

- Mental Stimulation and Stability – Consistent exercise can help improve your mental stability and support optimal cognitive function. According to the U.S. National Library of Medicine, exercise can reduce such negative mental conditions as anxiety, depression and mood swings while improving self-esteem. Following the minimum recommendations for exercise can improve your alertness and performance on your job as well as your ability to perform those minor tasks around the house.

How much physical activity is enough?

For those who doesn't engage in any physical activity and stay inactive for most part of the day, any form of regular exercise, however little would be enough. Whereas there are no strict routines that should be adhered to with reference to physical activities, different levels of physical activities have been recommended by the Physical Activity Guidelines for Americans. For instance, one can engage in two sessions of moderate intensity aerobics for half an hour each week or one vigorous intensity aerobics for a quarter an hour weekly. Alternatively, one can decide to combine both two for better results.

Studies show that adults need at least 150 minutes of moderate-intensity physical activity each week in addition to muscle-strengthening activities. If activity is more vigorous in intensity, 75 minutes a week may be enough. You can also do a combination of moderate and vigorous activity. The idea is to move more and to make it fun. A brisk walk in the park, a fun Zumba class, biking or running are ideal ways to get your heart pumping and those calories burning.

Track Your Progress

Technology has made it simple to track your daily activity level. Some provide added bonuses with features for monitoring heart rate, sleep patterns tracking daily food intake, and more. If you buy a smart pedometer or fitness tracker like a Fitbit, chances are the device will encourage you to take 10,000 steps a day. Experts say that while 10,000 steps a day is a good number to reach, any amount of activity beyond what you're currently doing will likely benefit your health. So whether you use a wristband tracking device, an app on your phone, or some other equipment, tracking your progress can help keep you motivated in achieving your desired level of activity each day.

Movement is a medicine for creating change in a person's physical, emotional, and mental states.

~ Carol Welch

Chapter Six: Nurture Yourself

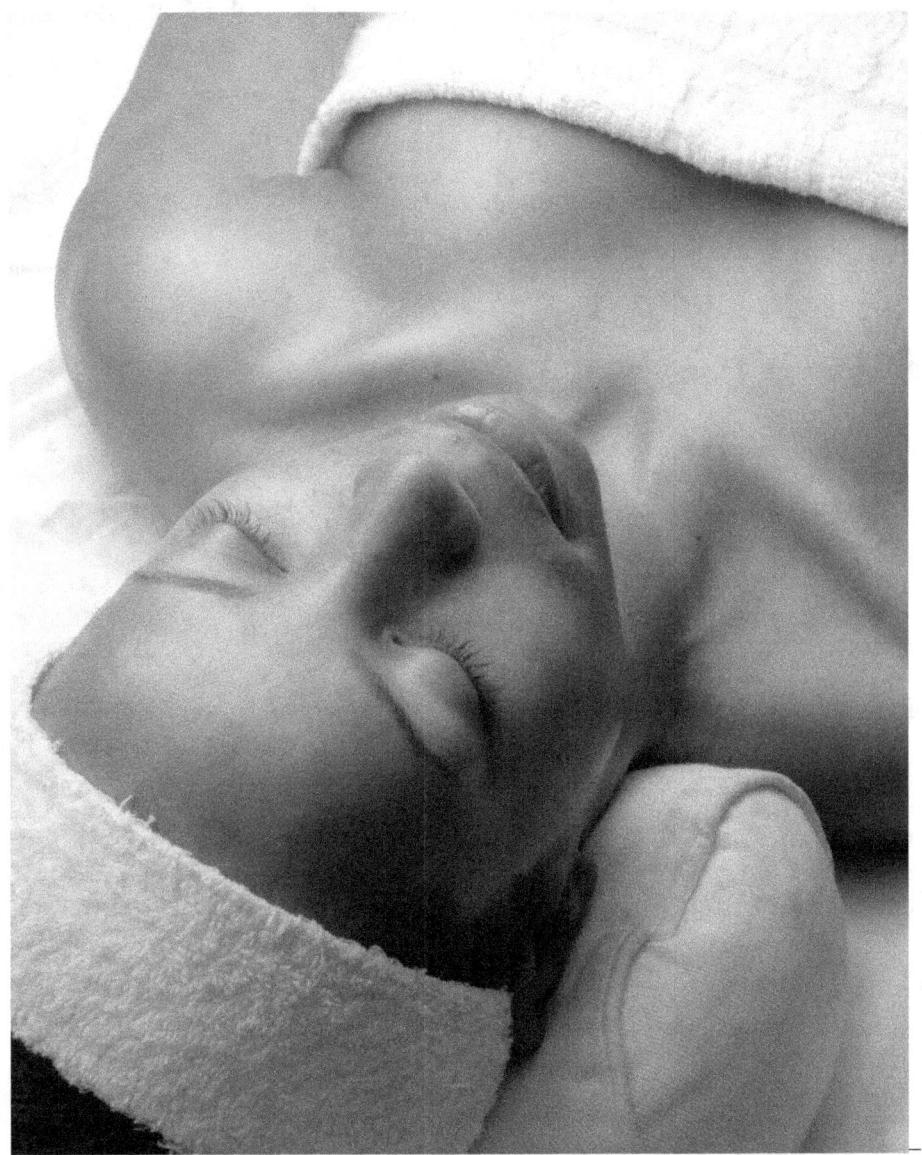

Reducing stress is vital for maintaining a healthy lifestyle. A majority of people are engrossed in the pursuit of different things of the modern world and it is very easy for someone to accumulate unprecedented levels of stress which can end up hurting them psychologically as well as physically. It thus becomes a matter of utmost importance to manage the stress levels lest you risk developing chronic stress which might have far reaching consequences to your body.

Physical effects of stress

The physical effects of stress become evident when stress is allowed to accumulate to higher levels within the body. It is also important to remember that when stress reaches chronic levels, it becomes the number one risk factor for conditions such as heart attack and cancer. The accumulation of stress in the body makes muscles to get tensed and as a result, they will react by triggering unwanted conditions such as migraines, headaches amongst others. Stress will also interfere with the digestive system and result in problems like nausea, constipation, heartburn, and vomiting.

Psychological effects of stress

Other than the physical effects, stress also leads to a number of emotional and mental conditions such as depression, panic attacks, phobia, anxiety etc. Stress will also make an individual to lose focus, have difficulty in making decisions as well as hamper their memory. Change in mood is another psychological effect of stress and it can lead to the development of feelings of anger, insecurity, lack of patience etc. Due to these physical and psychological effects of stress, it becomes important for every individual to avoid getting stressed as much as possible.

Center yourself

You can handle whatever tough situations you encounter with grace and wisdom. The key to doing so is keeping yourself centered in love and firmly grounded in your space – with your boundaries held securely about you. Centering yourself means to have a reference point, a place to come back to when life and emotions and stress push you off balance.

It can be as easy as taking a deep breath, a moment of being totally present to the physical sensation of the nourishing air flowing into your cells, the peacefulness in your heart, the momentary quiet of your busy mind. It can be a time of contemplation or prayer, song or dance. The beauty of a sunset, a butterfly, a child's face. A feeling of gratitude, like a smile that starts in your heart and spreads through your whole being and shifts you right back into your center.

Centering and grounding yourself are processes that should be practiced – ideally multiple times throughout the day to effectively manage stress. Benefits of this practice can improve your health greatly since some aliments in the body are stress related. Health benefits include:

Enhances emotional balance – centering yourself can cleanse your emotion of the bad memories which are replaced by good thoughts of freedom and abundance. During the process, unhealthy emotional states and neurosis get cured leaving the individual with a better emotional balance.

Improved immunity –When practiced regularly, they reduce the recurrence of breast cancer and they also boost the production of natural killer cells among the elderly thus improve their resistance to the development of cancerous tumors.

Lower blood pressure – centering yourself has been proven to reduce the body's response to stress hormones as well as to blood pressure. Besides, patients who consistently practices meditation and relaxation have been reported to have low blood pressure.

Anti-inflammatory – inflammation which leads to other serious conditions like arthritis, heart condition and asthma has a direct correlation with stress. Centering yourself can be used to reduce the levels of stress as you relax and allow your mind to release whatever anxiety or debilitating thoughts that triggered the stress. Relaxing in general is an effective form of therapy to reduce inflammation because it hinders the accumulation of stress in the body.

Simple ways on how to relax

There are several ways to meditate and achieve relaxation though a majority of people always think of yoga as the only method. Below are some simple tips on how to achieve relaxation in a very short period of time-:

➢ Meditate – this does not require you to go to the beach or some mountainous region to achieve. Simply find a silent and comfortable spot, concentrate on your breathing pattern then focus on your worries and anxiety and see them start to disappear.

➢ Lay your head on a pillow – a short nap in the middle of the day can work wonders towards making you relax but you might get fired when you do this in the office. Simply find a soft pillow or cushion, lay your head, close your eyes and visualize the pillow to be like a sponge absorbing all your fears and worries. Do this for about five minutes.

➢ Progressive relaxation – in this method, you tense muscles in one body part in a bid to attain a state of calmness. Do this each at a time for as many muscles as you possibly can.

➢ Journaling – putting down the accounts of your life is also a great way to relax. This is recommended at night before you go to bed as you will get a chance to go through the happenings of the day and identify particular changes you can make for better results tomorrow.

Nourishing yourself in a way that helps you blossom in the direction you want to go is attainable, and you are worth the effort.

~Deborah Day

Chapter Seven: Get Enough Sleep

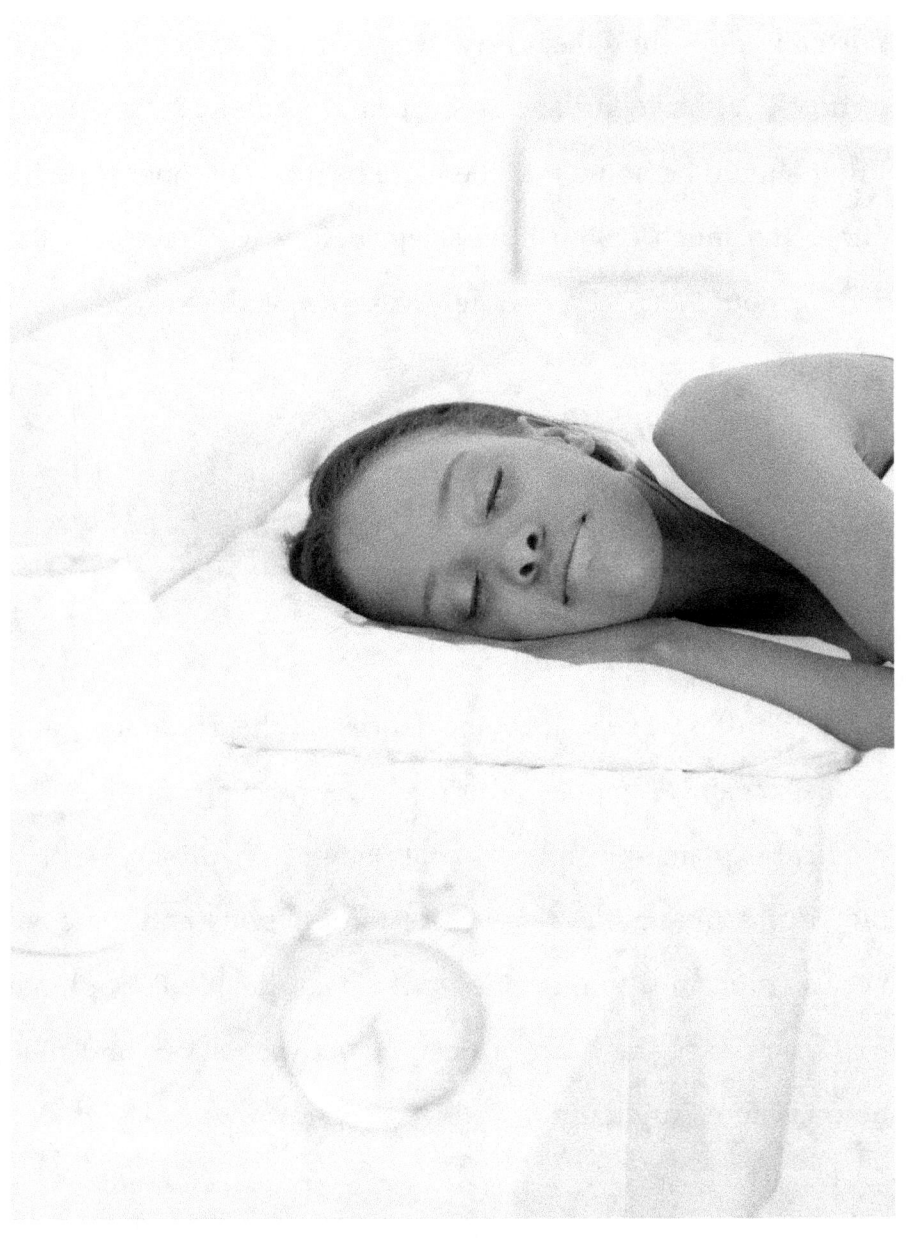

To some of us, sleep is just another routine yet to others, bedtime is their most adored moment of the day and they wish that morning would not come as quickly as it normally does. In either case, sleep remains to be an integral part of healthy living and in ensuring a good quality of life. But it should be noted that there are health consequences with either too much or too little sleep. Before we delve into the right amount of sleep, below are some of the reasons why sleep in important.

Benefits of adequate night rest

Sleep Enhances heart health

Studies reveal that incidences of heart attacks and strokes mainly happen during the morning hours. The medical explanation to this is that lack of sleep increases the blood pressure and levels of cholesterol in body and these are very significant when it comes to the heart health. For optimal performance of the heart, a sleep of between seven and nine hours is necessary daily.

Stress reduction

Sleep deprivation makes the body produce stress hormones which leads to the accumulation of stress in the body. Adequate sleep on the other hand inhibits the production of this hormone hence playing a crucial role in keeping the blood pressure in check as well as other related health conditions.

Increases alertness

When you get adequate sleep at night, you can expect to stay more active and alert as opposed to when you are deprived of sleep. You can also expect to stay more focused and have better judgment while going about your routine throughout the day.

Enhance the immune system

When you sleep, the body gets adequate time to produce new cells and repair those that have been damaged as a result of stress, free radicals, ultraviolet rays and the like. Adequate sleep improves your immune system thereby making you more resistant to diseases.

How much sleep is enough?

I often hear people say they can function on four to six hours of sleep each night, but research shows that adults who get fewer than seven hours of sleep – whether for just one night or over the course of days, week, or months – have more difficulty concentrating and more mood problems than people who sleep between seven to nine hours.

The amount of sleep needed is dependent mainly upon age. Children require more sleep than adults. According to the National Sleep Foundation Scientific Advisory Council, newborns require anywhere from 14 - 17 hours each day. This number declines as children mature with the average number being between 10 – 12 hours at age six. After becoming a young adult, the recommended sleep range is between 7-9 hours and remains the same until age 64.

Older adults (65+) may get fewer hours of sleep than when they were younger. As people age they tend to have a harder time falling asleep and more trouble staying asleep than when they were younger. It is a common misconception that sleep needs decline with age. Changes in the patterns of our sleep occur as we age. This may contribute to sleep problems, but the recommended amount of sleep remains the same.

How to prepare for a quality night rest

Getting a quality night sleep will allow you to be more refreshed and energized in the morning. First, create a relaxing serene atmosphere free from noise, light, and other distractions. Condition your mind so that it knows that this is a place where you sleep. Set a regular time for going to bed so your body will always signal sleep hormones naturally at the same time. Limit the amount of electronic devices used prior to going to bed, such as television, laptop, radio, cell phones, and other devices. Also, avoid caffeine and drinking too many liquids in the evening. To improve your sleep quality, do the following before retiring to bed:

- Dim the lights and switch off any sounds since light and sound will keep you more alert and make it difficult to fall asleep.
- Have your last meal at least three hours before bedtime so that most of the digestion is done by the time you go to bed.
- Clear your mind of any clutter that might make it difficult for you to get a sound sleep.
- Make sleep a priority.

Sleep is that golden chain that ties health and our bodies together.

~Thomas Dekker

Chapter Eight: Enjoy Your Life

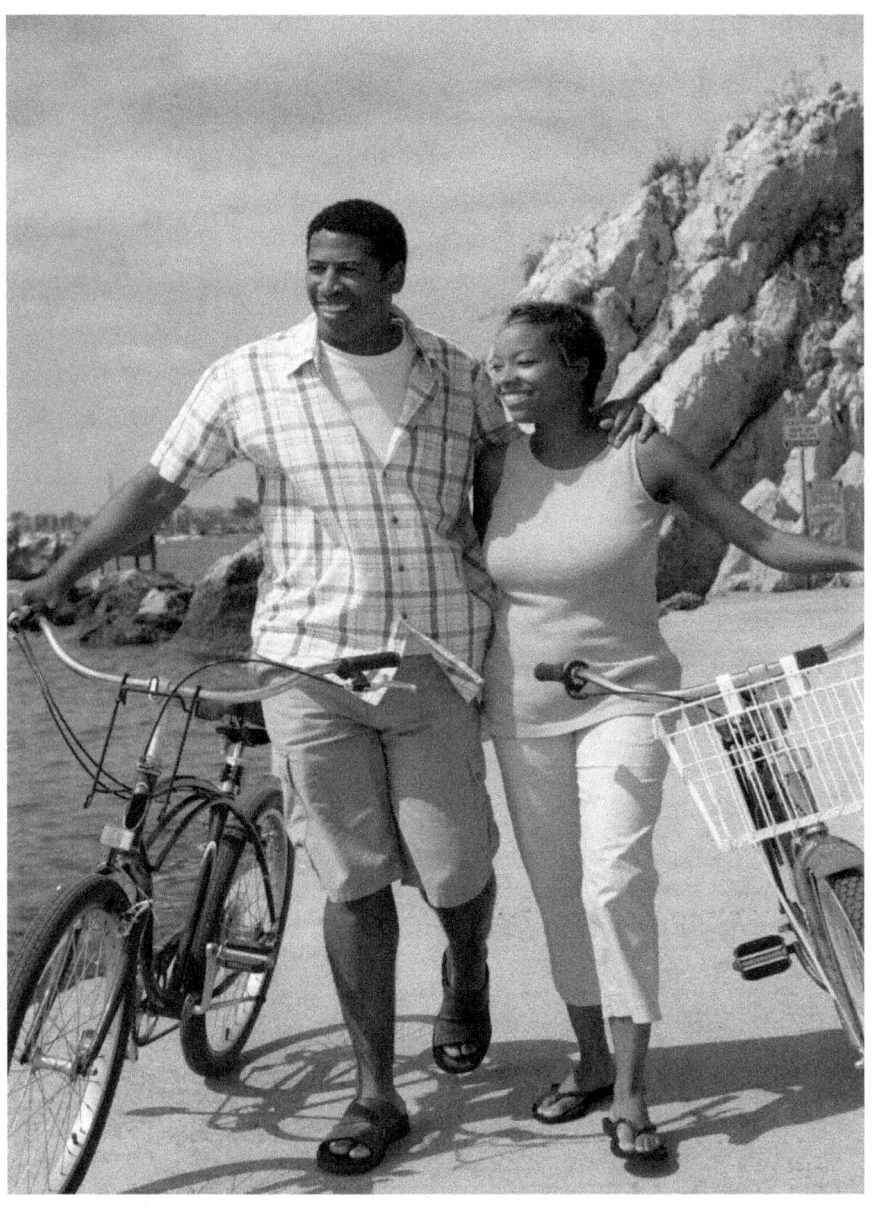

The secret to living a purposeful more meaningful life is learning to do what you love while creating great relationships along the way. It's taking time to breathe paying close attention to life's special moments. When was the last time you did something you really enjoyed? What are you most passionate about? What would you do more of if you could change your life right now? What would it take to fulfill your lifelong dream?

Surprisingly, some people never learn how to fully enjoy their lives. There is a misconception that in order to be happy we must attain a certain level. Enjoying your life has more to do with the journey rather than the destination. Happiness is not acquiring things or reaching a certain level in a career or in life or having an influential status. Happiness comes from within when we make a decision to be happy. It's really a mindset with our will and emotions following suit in agreement. Life is a present that must be unwrapped every day.

Life will present some things that are pleasant and some things that are not. Nevertheless, It is what we choose to do with what we've been dealt that matter most. Enjoying life is learning to make lemonade from lemons. Perhaps you've heard this phrase before.

Live Your Passion

Are you living out what you're passionate about? Here's how you can know. Does what you do fill your cup? Are you truly satisfied? Does it keep you up at night? Could you see yourself doing this for the rest of your life? Do you never tire of it? If your response is not yes to all of these questions then you may not have found your passion just yet. Life is too short to not enjoy your life by doing what you love and being compensated for it. You just have to take time to figure out what it is. It is usually so simple that it may be overlooked.

Here are a few questions to help you hone in on your passion. "If you could do anything you want and I mean anything, what would it be?" "What do you wish you could do?" "What do you find yourself doing all the time that comes natural to you?" "What do others say that you are really good at?" Pondering these questions will help start the process of identifying your passion. It may take time to really get to the core answers to these questions. So do not rush through this process.

Look for consistent themes that surface in your mind as you think through the questions. Write down every word or phrase that comes to mind. There is no wrong answer. Each word or phrase is needed to reveal your true passion. Once you think you have a clear picture of your passion then take the next step which is to explore what living this passion would look like. This is the visionary process. From there setting goals to realize the vision are the "next steps" towards living your passion.

Create Great Relationships!

Everything we do is connected to relationships. Whether its work, business, community, ministry or family – we develop relationships in various aspects of our lives because relationships are essential to overall wellbeing. We cannot survive without relationships – it's a primary food. Primary foods such as relationships, a fulfilling career, regular physical activity, and a spiritual practice are things that feed your soul and satisfy your hunger for life.

When primary food is balanced and satiating, your life feeds you, making what you eat secondary. The quality of these relationships explains a lot about the quality of a person's life and his or her health. What's important is to cultivate relationships that are healthy and support your individual needs, wants, and desires.

In any relationship you need boundaries. Personal boundaries are the limits we set in relationships that allow us to protect ourselves. Boundaries come from having a good sense of our own self-worth. They make it possible for us to separate our own thoughts and feelings from those of others and to take responsibility for what we think, feel and do.

Boundaries allow us to celebrate our own uniqueness. Intact boundaries are flexible - they allow us to get close to others when it is appropriate and to maintain our distance when we might be harmed by getting too close. Good boundaries protect us from abuse and pave the way to developing healthy relationships. They also help us take care of ourselves.

Good relationships are more than something we want—it's something we need to be our happiest, healthiest, most productive selves. But at home or work, supportive, fulfilling relationships don't come automatically. They take an investment in time and energy as well as social skills that can be learned. So be open as you meet people along life's journey. You never know when a great relationship may form.

Don't Sweat the Small Stuff

How often have we spent far too much time getting worked up over the smallest things? It seems as if almost everyone these days are walking around with elevated emotions that are just waiting to be triggered.

Some people take life's small slights and setbacks with a shrug, while others freak out, blow up, or fly off the proverbial handle in a loud huff or with silent seething. One thing for sure, stress is evident everywhere in our fast-paced world. It comes in many forms and enters our lives through a multitude of channels, which can become a mental, emotional, or physical strain if we're not careful.

A study shows that there's more stress in people's lives today than 25 years ago. As a matter of fact, the analysis indicates an increase of 18% for women and 24% for men from 1983 to 2009, according to researchers at Carnegie Mellon University in Pittsburgh, who analyzed data from more than 6,300 people.

Some lucky people are actually born with personalities that make them worry less, but what about the rest of us? We all feel stress from time to time and often suffer the results of it in some way or another, but how can we deal with such a pervasive force?

Here are a Five Tips to help you Balance Your Life:

1. **Prioritize Things.** So often we lose focus of what is really important. That's because we busy ourselves with things that seem right-to-do, but are not always beneficial. Avoid overloading yourself with menial tasks that still your precious time. Use the "Big Rocks" principle to prioritize your life. Identify the top 5 things that are important to you. Identify daily actions that include those priorities. When you focus on what is important first, the rest somehow all fits in.

2. **Use a schedule. Create a Plan.** I use a weekly schedule to plan each week. It includes time for appointments, exercising, quiet time, family time, fun time, and more. Using a schedule allows me to plan ahead to be more efficient with my time and energy. There is nothing more frustrating than missing opportunities because of lack of planning and then later stressing about it.

3. **Journal** – Writing can be very therapeutic. Something magical happens when you put your thoughts on paper. Journaling will allow you to declutter your mind by removing negative thoughts and stimulating new positive thoughts. I like early morning journaling when my thoughts are the clearest before the thoughts of the day settle in.

Countless times while journaling I have found solutions to problems and have come up with new ideas and new perspectives. But what I like most about journaling is being able to see personal growth. That in itself is worth more than its weight in gold.

4. **Practice Self-Care.** Taking care of yourself is essential. Most people have to practice self-care because so often their focus is on looking after others while neglecting themselves. In order to be of service to others we have to fill our cup first. This is where genuine acts of kindness come from – the place of wholeness.

Start carving out one hour per day to do something you really love. It could be a stroll in the park, hanging out with friends, pampering yourself at a spa, or simply cuddling up to read a good book.

However you spend this time is up to you as long as you are intentionally caring for your physical, mental, and emotional needs.

5. **Eat for better energy.** The foods we eat play an intricate role in our energy levels and our mood. Not surprisingly, vegetables, fruits, whole grains, high-fiber foods, and lean meats are high-level foods and are best at keeping energy levels up. Whereas low-level foods such as processed foods, fast foods, and junk foods zap energy levels, stimulate cravings, and increase stress. This later result in weight gain and fatigue. So be good to yourself and eat SMART.

Life is a present – unwrap it every day.

~Coach Denise

Other Books by the Author

1. Rejuvenate Your Health With 8 Simple Steps

2. Ohhmazing Wellness: Shift Your Vision and Create the Healthy & Happy Lifestyle You Deserve

3. My Life Healthy "Interactive" Wellness Journal

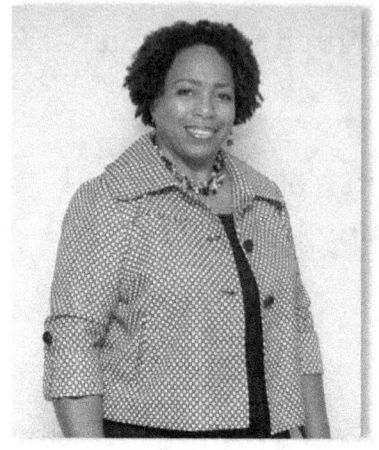

Denise N. Simpson is an influential leader in the field of health and wellness. She is Founder and CEO of My Life Healthy! with Denise, LLC, a company that is committed to cultivating health and wellness. Coach Denise is a highly trained Certified Holistic Health Practitioner through the American Association of Drugless Practitioners as well as a Certified Personal Trainer. She has studied over 100 dietary theories, practical lifestyle management techniques, and innovative coaching methods with some of the world's top health and wellness experts, including Dr. Andrew Weil, Dr. Deepak Chopra, Dr. Annmarie Colbin and Dr. Mark Hyman.

Coach Denise is also co-author to the International Best Seller anthology book *Ohhmazing Wellness: Shift Your Vision and Create the Healthy & Happy Lifestyle You Deserve*. She holds both, a Bachelor of Science and Masters of Public Administration degree from Florida State University. Coach Denise is married to her amazing husband Dennis of over 30 years, is mother to 3 remarkable adults and "Grammy" to 5 wonderful grandchildren.

Are you curious about how Coach Denise's wellness & lifestyle coaching can help you?
Contact her at: CoachDenise@MyLifeHealthy.com
For more information about My Life Healthy with Denise, LLC visit the website:

www.MyLifeHealthy.com

Follow Me on Social Media:

Facebook: @coachdenisesimpson

Instagram: @coachdenisesimpson

Twitter:@ MyCoachDenise

www.ingramcontent.com/pod-product-compliance
Lightning Source LLC
Chambersburg PA
CBHW071228280526
45787CB00002B/842